reduce craving

20 QUICK TECHNIQUES

KATRIN SCHUBERT, MD

Hazelden
Publishing

Hazelden Publishing
Center City, Minnesota 55012
hazelden.org/bookstore

Library of Congress Cataloging-in-Publication Data
Names: Schubert, Katrin, 1960- author.
Title: Reduce craving : 20 quick techniques /
Katrin Schubert, MD.
Description: Center City, Minnesota : Hazelden
Publishing, 2016. | Series:
    5-minute first aid for the mind
Identifiers: LCCN 2015038202 | ISBN 9781616496371
(paperback)
Subjects: LCSH: Compulsive behavior—Alternative
treatment.
Classification:
LCC RC533.S37 2016 | DDC 616.85/84—dc23
LC record available at http://lccn.loc.gov/2015038202

20 19 18 17 16   1 2 3 4 5 6

Cover design: Kathi Dunn, Dunn + Associates
Interior illustrations: David Spohn
Author photo: Deb Stagg
Developmental editor: Sid Farrar
Production editor: Heather Silsbee

To Gerda and Philipp

CONTENTS

Introduction

Many years ago I had the pleasure of teaching an ear-acupuncture program to addiction counselors who worked at the publicly funded Street Health Clinic. The counselors worked with people addicted to street drugs, and the program was designed to treat cravings and detoxification. The clinic's clientele consisted of folks whose hard lives were imprinted on their faces, their demeanor, their dress, and their speech. As part of the training, the counselors had invited a number of their clients for a trial treatment at the clinic.

One woman in particular stood out to me. She sat with her friend, the two of them looking older than their age, huddled together for support. After her treatment, the woman took a long, slow breath and relaxed, her eyes softening. "This is the most peace of mind I have felt in decades," she said.

From that moment on, I felt even more inspired than before to self-empower people—not just addicts, but all people whose cravings are interfering with their ability to live a fulfilling life—by giving them techniques they can use on themselves and on their friends to find some solace. I believe that every person should have some tools at their fingertips that enable them to help themselves in moments of need, and that one moment of relief will add to the next, allowing them a glimpse of the possibilities ahead.

Understanding Cravings

Most of us experience cravings for pleasurable things such as food, a drink, shopping, or sex. That doesn't mean we are addicted to those substances or behaviors. Cravings are natural and only become a problem when we're unable to control them and they negatively affect our well-being and quality of life. This can happen on a spectrum, from

- periodic cravings that we give in to every so often resulting in few or no problems, to

- compulsions that we surrender to on a regular enough basis that we experience some negative consequences (such as weight gain from eating too many sweets or maxing out our credit card from overspending), to

- full addiction, when the craving for the substance or behavior takes over our lives and we need professional help.

There are many reasons we experience cravings and feel the need to give in to them. A craving can feel like a physical need at times, and sometimes the body is expressing some biological deficiency. Usually, however, our cravings arise out of psychological distress and the need to "medicate" uncomfortable feelings such as anxiety, anger, boredom, sadness, or loneliness.

One thing, however, is always true: when we have an uncontrollable need to indulge to the point that our behavior becomes a bad habit or full-blown addiction, we always feel cut off from our inner self, from the best that we can be and the full manifestation of our talents. We feel fragmented and experience a void we think we have to fill in order to feel whole again. In many ways, we in the Western world are an addicted society. Our fast-paced and ungrounded lifestyle messes with our brains, pushing us to indulge in mood-altering behaviors to soothe the eternal and instinctual search for fullness.

This book is designed to be used as a first-aid kit of techniques that can self-empower you to find more natural, healthful ways to soothe yourself. Whether you are in active counseling, a recovery program, or just want to instill healthier habits into your life, these techniques can be a valuable additional source of support. They can serve as a Band-Aid for the moment until you can get more support if you need it, and if used over time, they can help promote balance in your life. However, this book does not replace rehabilitation, counseling, or medical treatment. Only you can decide how much more assistance you need to reduce or free yourself from cravings.

How to Use This Book

You may want to work through the twenty techniques in order, or you may choose to spontaneously open the book to techniques that look appealing and try those first. No matter which approach you fancy, I recommend you try every technique at least once, settle on your favorite ones, and turn them into habits. The more you practice the techniques, the more you will remember them later on when you feel the need for support.

Each of the techniques collected in this book takes approximately five minutes to do. You may decide to apply a technique for a longer time or repeat the techniques several times each day. Some of the exercises take a little more time to prepare. But once you have spent ten to fifteen minutes making one of the lists or trying a more involved technique, you will be able to apply them in five minutes as they will become second nature.

Cravings are often related to stress, and you'll find a few of the techniques in this book are also recommended in another 5-Minute First Aid for the Mind title, *Relieve Stress*.

The 5-Minute First Aid for the Mind techniques have been tested and applied by thousands of people with good results. I have collected them and used them with my clients over the past twenty-some years as well as test driven them myself.

May they help you on your journey!

• • •

Part I:

The Techniques

Happy and Sad and Lonely
SOOTHING GRIEF AND LIFTING SPIRITS

Anne felt a terrible void after her husband had fallen ill and died within a year. It all seemed to happen so suddenly, and Anne felt as if someone had switched off the light in her life. She did not find pleasure in the activities she had previously enjoyed, and life seemed dull. Anne started drinking habitually in the evenings to overcome her loneliness, and within a short while alcohol became a daytime companion as well. Anne reached out for professional help to overcome her dependence. In addition, she used acupressure on her own and found that it made a big difference in her well-being.

•

Grieving and feeling low in spirits can lead to cravings, as we use substances and behaviors to ease emotional pain and fill an aching void within us.

Acupressure is a complementary health care modality based on the ancient Chinese understanding that the body contains a life energy which circulates through specific channels in the body. These channels, called meridians, relate to organs, body parts, and the central nervous system. By massaging acupressure points that are scattered along the meridians, the energy flow within the point and meridian can be improved and self-healing can be promoted. Balancing acupressure points can benefit the body and mind on many levels. Both acupressure and acupuncture are powerful healing modalities.

This technique uses two powerful acupressure points that can help to uplift us and elevate our mood.

Stimulating the acupressure point called CV 17 helps to relieve grief, open our chest to deeper breathing, and lift the weight of sadness, a feeling that often leads to cravings for mood-altering substances and behaviors to artificially lift our spirits. The point lies right in the middle of your breastbone and, if tender to touch, is an excellent area for a massage. The beauty of this point is that we can massage it while watching TV, reading a book, or just hanging out.

Stimulating the point called Li4 (Large Intestine 4) can help to relieve any distress in the head and brain, from headaches and toothaches to mental states of sadness and discontent. It is also useful for relieving stress, a common trigger for cravings, and I included it in my book *Relieve Stress: 20 Quick Techniques* as well. Many of my clients have reported feeling better, more energetic, and more positive after massaging that point.

HOW TO DO IT

The acupressure point CV 17 is located in the center of the breastbone on your chest. If you feel tenderness

ACUPRESSURE POINT CV 17 ON CHEST

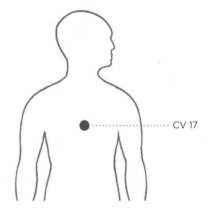

CV 17

Massage this point for three to five minutes.

slightly higher or lower than the described area, follow that sensation and massage the most tender point.

Use your index and middle fingers of one hand to massage CV 17. You may want to apply a small circular motion while using just enough pressure to feel some tenderness. Massage this point for three to five minutes and repeat several times per day for the most benefit.

Stimulating CV 17 can help to open your chest and improve your breathing, and can reduce the pressure on the chest often experienced when grieving. You may notice a lessening of sadness. The translation of the Chinese name for this acupressure point means "sea of tranquility" because of its ability to calm upset emotions.

Li4 is an acupressure point located in the fleshy, muscular part of the hand between the thumb and index finger. You may notice that this area feels tender or achy when you massage it. This is a good sign, and it means you should work it for several minutes.

It is best to massage this area between your thumb and index finger from both sides, gently pinching the palm side and the back of your hand at the same time.

Massage each hand for three to five minutes and repeat if you wish. Over time this acupressure point may be less tender, indicating that you are in better balance. Acupressure on Li4 can help to lift your spirits, get you out of the blues, and help you avoid giving in to cravings for mood-altering substances or behaviors that have medicated those feelings in the past. As an added bonus, it can ease headaches and colds, stimulate your immune system, and make you feel happier.

HAPPY POINT ACUPRESSURE

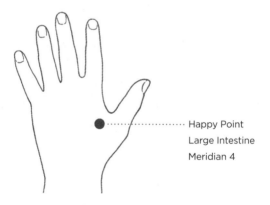

Happy Point
Large Intestine
Meridian 4

Massage each hand for three to five minutes.

Women for Sobriety and Men for Sobriety

THE NEW LIFE ACCEPTANCE PROGRAM

I was first introduced to Women for Sobriety (WFS) by Janine, a client of mine who worked as a guard in a maximum security prison. Having witnessed extreme violence among the inmates, she suffered from nightmares and had made it a habit to drink a bottle of wine to "soothe her nerves" almost every evening after work. The thirteen statements of WFS helped her deal with her cravings and recover.

·

Allison reads the thirteen statements of Women for Sobriety almost every day. She then chooses one statement to ponder for the day, but without fail she will have forgotten it within an hour. Even though she does not actively remember it during her day, she has noticed over a few weeks that many issues have just fallen away from her daily life. She feels more positive about herself, and she recognizes that the thirteen statements have been life-altering for her on a deeper level, shifting her harsh self-judgment to a gentle acceptance. When she notices that she is engaging in negative thoughts about herself, one of her triggers for cravings, she is able to turn them around more quickly and more effectively. While Allison would have been very self-critical in the past for forgetting the statement after she reads it, she now realizes that her mind has shifted to be more embracing of her perceived shortcomings.

·

Sometimes it can seem that men and women come from different planets. While we are waiting for scientific proof of that notion, many of us are convinced it is true. WFS was developed by one woman with the understanding that women usually have different requirements and a different psychological makeup than men do.

Jean, the creator of WFS, understood that women generally have the "need to nurture feelings of self-value and self-worth and the desire to discard feelings of guilt, shame, and humiliation." The organization's New Life Program is based on thirteen positive statements that help women overcome substance use issues. I have found that using these statements can reduce craving, whether it's associated with an addiction or it's just causing distress in one's life. These positive statements are effective on their own when cravings occur or can be used in conjunction with a Twelve Step or other recovery program. They have also proven effective for men as applied by the more recently developed Men for Sobriety.

HOW TO DO IT

Take a few minutes in the morning to read and ponder the thirteen statements, and then pick out one that speaks to you and make it the theme of your day. This means that you can call forth that statement in your mind when you encounter feelings or a situation that triggers a craving for an unhealthy substance or behavior.

I posted these statements on my refrigerator door. On days when I do not have enough time for my morning reading, I will pick one statement while opening the fridge to look for my breakfast.

If you don't have an addiction, you may remove the words "life-threatening" from the first statement and replace the word "disease" with "craving." I am certain that you will find these statements helpful no matter your gender.

NEW LIFE PROGRAM
13 POSITIVE STATEMENTS

1. I have a life-threatening problem that once had me.

   I now take charge of my life and my disease. I accept the responsibility.

2. Negative thoughts destroy only myself.

   My first conscious sober act must be to remove negativity from my life.

3. Happiness is a habit I will develop.

   Happiness is created, not waited for.

4. Problems bother me only to the degree I permit them to.

   I now better understand my problems and do not permit problems to overwhelm me.

5. I am what I think.

   I am a capable, competent, caring, compassionate woman/man.

6. Life can be ordinary or it can be great.
   Greatness is mine by a conscious effort.

7. Love can change the course of my world.
   Caring becomes all important.

8. The fundamental object of life is emotional and
   spiritual growth.
   Daily I put my life into a proper order,
   knowing which are the priorities.

9. The past is gone forever.
   No longer will I be victimized by the past.
   I am a new person.

10. All love given returns.
    I will learn to know that others love me.

11. Enthusiasm is my daily exercise.
    I treasure all moments of my new life.

12. I am a competent woman/man and have much
    to give life.
    This is what I am and I shall know it always.

13. I am responsible for myself and for my actions.
    I am in charge of my mind, my thoughts,
    and my life.

TECHNIQUE 3

The Brain in Your Toes
FOOT REFLEXOLOGY

Nicole checked her email and Facebook account every free minute she had. She used to read or talk with friends and family in the evening, but she had now become hooked on blogging until very late at night. It left her body tense and her mind tired and unsatisfied, yet she found it very difficult to resist the compulsion to go online and to break this pattern of behavior.

Nicole noticed that she felt much more grounded in her body and in the present moment when she started massaging her feet, particularly her toes and the space between them. It helped her to engage in meaningful interactions outside of the Internet, and she noticed that she felt happier and more connected to her real surroundings.

*

The soles of our feet contain nerve pathways that correspond with every organ, body part, and system in our body. These corresponding areas on the soles of our feet are called reflexes and the soles of the feet are considered a "reflex organ." We have many other reflex organs as well, which have similar energetic representations, such as the palms of our hands and the auricles, or external portion of our ears.

Foot reflexologists are health care practitioners who specialize in how our organs correspond with specific areas on the soles of our feet. They are trained in the art and science of reflexology to alleviate ailments by massaging our feet in just the right areas.

If you have never experienced a good foot massage, try massaging your feet yourself. It will likely produce a profound sense of relaxation, a bit of bliss, and maybe even some sound sleep if you do it before bedtime.

When you feel cranky and stressed and tempted to give in to your urges for mood-altering substances or behaviors, try massaging the trigger points on your feet described in this technique—it is a healthier fix that can change your mood for the better.

HOW TO DO IT

Sitting comfortably, rest your right foot above your left knee and turn the sole of your right foot upward so you can see the underside of your foot.

Start massaging your foot without using any lotion or oil. Use one or both thumbs to work the bottom of your foot, and make sure you massage the sides of the foot and the full length of each toe, including the tip. Vigorously massage the web between each toe.

The toes correspond to the brain and its glands; you are bound to find some tender spots in your toes as well as in many other parts of the soles of your feet. The same principle used in acupressure applies to reflexology as well: spend a good amount of time on the achy spots, as they indicate an imbalance. After massaging one spot for thirty seconds or so, you may realize that it is not nearly as sore as it was when you first started. That is a good sign!

When you are done, notice any changes you may be feeling in your body, your emotions, or your thoughts. Have your muscles relaxed? Has your face softened? Has your mood changed? Make a mental note of those things.

Now give your left foot the same treatment. Here are some areas to pay special attention to.

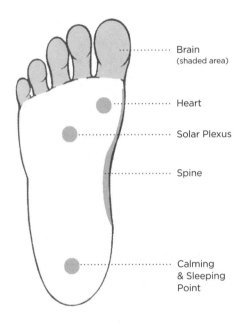

Brain
(shaded area)

Heart

Solar Plexus

Spine

Calming
& Sleeping
Point

Spend a good amount of time on the achy spots.

And here are the locations of some important corresponding organs and body parts.

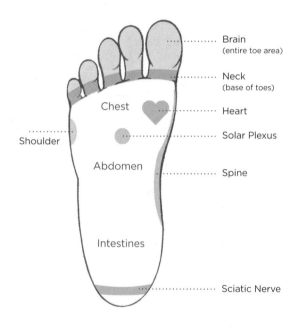

	Brain (entire toe area)
	Neck (base of toes)
Chest	Heart
Shoulder	Solar Plexus
Abdomen	Spine
Intestines	
	Sciatic Nerve

Areas of the foot correspond with every part of our body.

While the notion of reflex organs may sound far-fetched in our logical Western worldview, many an unfamiliar modality has been supported by sound scientific evidence. In the case of reflexology and energy medicine, having a positive experience with a treatment will win over the skeptical, logical brain. Try a good foot rub and then check in with yourself and evaluate whether you feel any different. Most people will notice an improved sense of well-being. Not every treatment or intervention, however, whether from Eastern medicine or Western medicine, will work for every person. Each of us has a unique body and mind, and some things work better for us than others. It's best to keep an open mind and continue to try new things, especially if, as in the case of foot reflexology, they've been proven to work for so many people!

Best Buddies

Omar says, "A number of my friends know that I am trying to quit smoking, and when I feel weak and just about to give in, I call one of my friends. It makes me feel so much better. It is good to know that I have friends who care about me. Talking to them reduces my sense of loneliness and helps me feel more connected to myself."

This exercise requires a little preparation, but once it is set up it can be done in a matter of minutes.

Nothing makes us feel better than loving contact with another human being. Think of the warm, fuzzy, and uplifted feeling you experience when you spend quality time with friends or family, even like-minded people you do not know very well. We have all experienced the opposite as well—the sense of frustration and emptiness after difficult interactions when we were unable to connect with someone in our hearts and minds.

When our minds are chewing on something or we have stumbled upon some pothole in the journey of life, nothing makes us feel better than being able to talk with someone who understands and can listen compassionately. Feeling accepted for who we are is our core longing, no matter how dysfunctional our insides feel. To get relief from cravings of any kind, it can be very helpful to find a like-minded and supportive buddy you can connect with. I suggest that you talk with someone you trust and who has your best interest at heart. The emphasis naturally is on *like-minded* and *supportive*.

This type of support is the strength of Alcoholics Anonymous (AA) and other similar programs, where members support each other and people can find extra help from their sponsors. The buddy system also works very well in scuba diving, and your adventure of dealing with cravings may at times feel like you're under water without oxygen. Thankfully, you don't need an air tank or oxygen mask to pull through; just call up your friends and talk when your cravings are about to drown you.

It's also a good idea to meet with your friends in person, but choose your venue wisely. Talking to your smoking friends at the bar while they are having a beer will not help you deal with your cravings when you are trying to quit smoking and drinking. Meeting your friend at the mall when you are trying to pay off your credit card debt is digging a trap for yourself.

This technique may entail making new friends or asking your existing ones to support you in helpful ways. It may mean creating new habits and choosing new surroundings for your friendships. There will be new friends for you when you make the decision to find them. Many of us already have a good friend, an understanding spouse, or a compassionate family member or coworker; many others will have to make new friends in order to meet their needs. Blogs, interest groups, and social clubs are excellent places to find new friends with similar interests. Thanks to the Internet, we don't always have to leave home—even though it is preferable to interact in person—in order to connect with someone on an emotional level.

Knowing the first cues that cause you to crave is very helpful in managing that craving. At the first signs of a trigger, connect with a supportive friend.

The sooner you can initiate this technique, the better the results.

HOW TO DO IT

Identify a small group of like-minded friends and enlist them to be your buddies in times of need. You may want to choose one as your special go-to person who can also take on more of a mentor role.

Spend a little time on this preparation before you are desperate for the next "fix" and you will be ready to use the technique as soon as an urge strikes:

1. Make a list of triggers that cause inconsolable yearnings and cravings for your unwanted behavior. You know yourself: observe which people, places, and things usually push you over the edge.

2. Make a list of people who you know will be supportive of you, and write down their phone numbers and email addresses. If you cannot think of anyone, seek out blogs, support groups, or help lines that will invite you in.

3. Make sure your potential buddies are willing to connect with you if you feel the need to do so.

Let them know what you will need from them when you call. You may just want them to listen without trying to fix your situation, or you may want to listen to their own personal wisdom.

4. It is a good idea to have more than one buddy so you don't wear out any one person when things get especially bumpy for you. Also, you may not always be able to reach one person, so having backup is important. Some therapists say that it takes seven friends to help someone through a life crisis.

List of triggers that cause cravings:

_____

_____

_____

_____

_____

_____

_____

Make a list of supportive people, with names and phone numbers, email addresses, and common interests (add chat-room usernames or blog addresses if available):

Name _____

Phone _____

Email _____

Common Interests _____

_____

_____

Username or Blog _____

Name _____

Phone _____

Email _____

Common Interests _____

_____

_____

Username or Blog _____

Name _____

Phone _____

Email _____

Common Interests _____

_____

_____

Username or Blog _____

Name _____

Phone _____

Email _____

Common Interests _____

_____

_____

Username or Blog _____

Name _____

Phone _____

Email _____

Common Interests _____

_____

_____

Username or Blog _____

Name _____

Phone _____

Email _____

Common Interests _____

_____

_____

Username or Blog _____

Name _____

Phone _____

Email _____

Common Interests _____

_____

_____

Username or Blog _____

Name _____

Phone _____

Email _____

Common Interests _____

_____

_____

Username or Blog _____

TECHNIQUE 5

Square Breathing

Cravings can keep our minds busy—very busy! Our thoughts can act like hamsters on a wheel, constantly running over the same ground. How exhausting this can be, and how tempting to give in!

Square breathing is a wonderful technique to give your mind a holiday from revolving thoughts. When I decide I need some square breathing, I can almost feel my brain relaxing and sighing a breath of relief, knowing it can get off the hamster wheel. My stress melts away.

It is also a fabulous technique to use when I have trouble falling asleep or when my mind awakens in the middle of the night whirling with thoughts. The square breathing technique is a favorite among my clients and friends.

HOW TO DO IT

Find a square or rectangular object in your surroundings. It can be a picture frame or door if you are indoors, or a car window, section of a sidewalk, or a
flower box if you are out in the city. Even the great
outdoors will offer squares or rectangles in the form
of stones, bushes, or fences.

Now move your eyes from the top left corner of
your box horizontally to the right side while inhaling.
This means you move in a clockwise fashion. Be
mindful to slow down your eye movements and
breath. Once you reach the upper right corner, move
your eyes downward in a very deliberate fashion

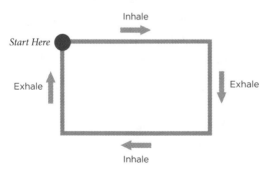

SQUARE BREATHING

while slowly exhaling. Breathe in along the bottom corner from right to left, and then breathe out from the bottom left upward to your starting point. Keep moving your eyes along the square or rectangle while slowing down your breath, inhaling along the top and bottom edges and exhaling along the sides. Ideally your out-breath should last as long as your in-breath. Breathe around the square for several rounds or two to five minutes, and repeat the exercise if you feel your uneasy thoughts returning. You may also want to change the direction of your eye movement to counterclockwise for added benefit.

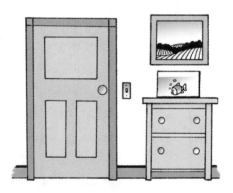

Find a square or rectangular object in your surroundings.

You may notice that your mind becomes occupied with moving your eyes from one corner to the next while synchronizing your breathing, leaving no "mind space" for anxious thoughts. You may feel a sense of calm, and it can help reset your nervous system. (This technique is also included in my book *Relieve Stress: 20 Quick Techniques*.)

TECHNIQUE 6

Tap, Tap, Tap Away
EMOTIONAL FREEDOM

Tapping is a psychological stress-relief technique that helps to reset your internal "thermostat" for mind-body health, thus reducing anxiety, a major trigger for cravings. Developed in the 1990s by Dr. Roger Callahan and Stanford graduate Gary Craig, tapping, or Emotional Freedom Technique (EFT), is based on the system of acupuncture. It involves finding an emotional trigger and using that trigger in an affirmative sentence. This is followed by a sequence of tapping on points that help with processing. The beauty of the system is that you can be very specific in what kind of stress and the resulting craving you want to reduce, and you can do it almost any place you find yourself.

Tapping helps us to cope with life's stressors by stimulating specific acupuncture points on the meridian system of the body. It has the remarkable ability to de-stress and relax us while improving our immune system at the same time. It can balance our autonomic nervous system, reduce cravings, and even reduce pain and fears. It is one of the most powerful self-help techniques I have come across.

Once you have learned this easy technique, you will be able to use it anytime and anywhere. You will learn to make your own custom-tailored stress-reduction statement and then tap on prescribed points with your fingertips. Most likely you will notice a remarkable decline in your overall stress level.

The first time you try tapping, it will likely take a little while to find the correct sequence of the tapping points. After one or two rounds, this technique should only take a few minutes.

HOW TO DO IT

Here are the three basic steps. You will then find an explanation of how exactly to do them.

1. Find your stress statement and rate your level of stress.

2. Voice your statement and goal.

3. Tap away your stress.

Here are the details:

1. Find your stress statement

Make a list of the things that are currently bothering you. Here are some examples:

- I am craving cake, chips, or ice cream.

- I want to smoke a cigarette right now.

- I am afraid of speaking at the meeting.

- I am angry with my sister-in-law and it is making me crave.

- I get anxious when my wife is intoxicated.

My stress statements:

_____

_____

_____

_____

_____

_____

_____

_____

Choose the statement that is bothering you the most and circle it. Rate the severity of that issue between 0 and 100 percent, and write down the percentage next to the statement.

2. Voice your statement and goal using the following format:

"Even though I _____ (fill in your stress statement here), I still deeply and completely love and accept myself."

Say this to yourself with conviction while you rub and wiggle the thumb and index finger of one hand on the inside ends of both collarbones. You should

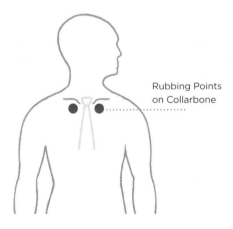

Rubbing Points
on Collarbone

have your thumb on one point and your index finger on the other so you are rubbing both point simultaneously. If you have trouble finding the correct points, imagine you are wearing a tie and put your thumb and index finger on either side of the bottom of the knot of the tie.

Here are some other examples:

"Even though I am angry with my parents for giving me a curfew, I still deeply and completely love and accept myself."

"Even though I am desperately wanting to eat this junk food, I still deeply and completely love and accept myself."

Fill in your own phrase:

"Even though I _____ , I still deeply and completely love and accept myself."

Declaring that we "deeply love ourselves" can be difficult and may act as its own kind of trigger for us. If you find it challenging to say this to yourself, you may want to shorten the sentence to "I still deeply and completely accept myself" and add the word "love" back in later when you feel more at ease with it.

For example:

"Even though I_____,
I still deeply and completely accept myself."

3. Tap away your stress

Tap with the index and middle fingers held together on these points on your head, face, and body as well as your hand while repeating your personal statement in your mind.

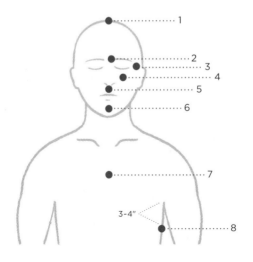

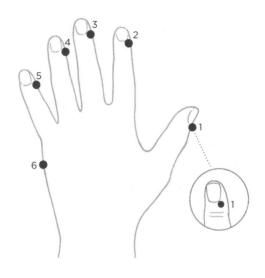

Tapping points on your hand

Note: The point on the fourth finger (the ring finger) is not part of the original EFT protocol. For ease of memorizing the sequence I have included tapping on the ring finger, and I am certain it will add to the benefit of the program.

Tap gently and rhythmically on each point for the length of a full, slow breath cycle in and out. It does not matter what side of the body you tap on or which hand you use, nor does it matter if you switch sides of the body in the middle of your tapping procedure. Just go ahead and tap without overthinking how accurate your tapping is. If you feel compelled to stay on one point for longer than one breath, listen to your inner voice and stay there until you feel something shifting; then move on to the next point.

When you are finished tapping all points, check whether your stress statement has lost some of its intensity. Has the percentage of your stress rating declined? If so, that would indicate the tapping is working for you. If it has not lessened at all after a few rounds of tapping, do not give up. You may have to revise your statement to be more accurate, or you may have to find a health care professional who can assist you in this process.

Tapping works for many situations in your life, not just reducing cravings, and you can do it anywhere at any time. Your stress levels should decrease with this technique as your brain lets go of more of its unhappy triggers.

Once you have done a few test runs, you can apply the tapping technique in just a couple of minutes.

Bonus Point

The tapping technique described here can significantly help put your mind at ease. Should you wish to make this technique even more beneficial, there is a bonus tapping point that can help to open the connection between the right and left hemispheres of your brain. Part 2 will tell you more about the science and benefits of the connected brain and how these techniques help to open the superhighway between your brain hemispheres, the famous corpus callosum.

Once you have finished your round of tapping as described previously, loosely hold your index and middle fingers together and tap on the back of your hand about two inches below the web between your ring and little fingers.

While tapping the spot on the back of your hand, do the following for about five to fifteen seconds each:

1. Close your eyes.
2. Open your eyes.

3. Look down to your right without turning your head.

4. Look down to the left without turning your head.

5. Roll your eyes slowly clockwise.

6. Roll your eyes slowly counterclockwise.

7. Hum a tune.

8. Count backward from ten to one.

9. Hum a tune.

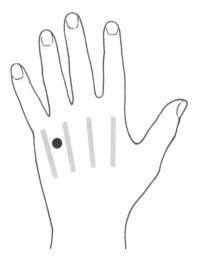

A bonus tapping point on your hand

Random Acts of Kindness

*Piglet noticed that even though he
had a Very Small Heart, it could hold a
rather large amount of Gratitude.*

—A.A. MILNE, *WINNIE-THE-POOH*

When we are sitting around with nothing better to do than think about our cravings and are tempted to give in to our substance or behavior of choice, there is nothing better than springing into action and donating some of our time to help out someone else.

Committing random acts of kindness is a spontaneous way to take our mind off ourselves and focus on something positive. Small gestures of kindness without expecting anything in return are very rewarding and can shift our state of mind. It can stop the slippery slope of caving in to our unhealthy choices by putting our feet back on the ground.

Your random acts of kindness can be extended to anyone, whether you know the person or not.

(Needless to say, you want to respect the recipient's privacy and not overstep boundaries.) Kindness can make a big difference in someone's life. Never underestimate the large impact of a small gesture.

HOW TO DO IT

- Greet people with a smile.
- Help someone load their car.
- Pick up someone's dropped belonging and make friendly eye contact.
- Walk someone's dog.
- Make a meal or mow the lawn for someone.
- Take out the trash without being asked.
- Reach out with kind words to someone.
  (For example: "It's always so good to see you."
  "I really enjoy spending time with you."
  "Please let me know if there is anything I
   can help you with.")
- Other acts of kindness:

  _____

  _____

It is best to pick an act of kindness that is meaningful to the person and that unburdens their life, even in a very small way.

Unlike Technique 13, The Secret of Service, random acts of kindness need no preparation or long-term commitment. They can happen on the spot and may require only a few seconds or minutes of your time.

TECHNIQUE 8

Cleanse Your Cravings Away

Alessandra has a habit of snacking in the evening. The last few years she has felt more general anxiety. The tenser she feels, the more she wants to eat chips and cookies. The head massage described here has helped to reduce her tension, and when she feels more mellow she is able to relax in the evening without the compulsion to eat unhealthy foods.

·

I have often felt that counseling 101 should be mandatory training for hairdressers. There is hardly anything more relaxing than having our hair shampooed. The fingertips of the stylist massage our head until our entire being enters a state of serenity.

In this relaxed state, we might then share with the stylist the problems and challenges we are currently facing in life. This in turn increases our self-awareness and mental-emotional processing, therefore releasing some of the "pressure cooker" thoughts that drive our unhealthy behaviors.

Having our scalp massaged with firm pressure on reflex and acupressure points helps us reach a different, calmer, more content state of mind. In that state we do not care as much about the nitty-gritty details of our lives, including our cravings. We are too at ease to give in to our "fixes."

The good news is that we do not have to train as hairstylists in order to enter this peaceful state of mind. With a little guidance, we can find the magical trigger points and give ourselves a good head and body massage that may shift our mind away from pursuing an unhealthy indulgence.

HOW TO DO IT

Massage your scalp

Spread the fingers of your cupped hands while gently maintaining some tension in them. Now place all fingertips on your scalp and make small, circular massaging motions. Start well above your ears, exploring your entire head with your fingers—a road trip around your skull, so to speak. Feel the small mountains and valleys and the soft or tense muscles with your circulating fingertips. Move your fingers

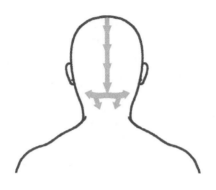

Massage paths on back of head

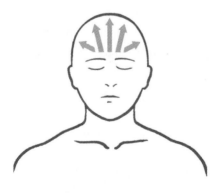

Massage paths on top of head

back toward the nape of your neck and keep massaging. Explore all the soft and bony spots, and linger with your massaging fingertips wherever it feels tender. Make sure you move your fingers to the midline at the top of your head and apply good pressure. Include your temples as well; the temple muscle works hard when you feel stressed and will welcome a little R & R.

How do you feel now compared to a few minutes ago?

Add to your technique by cleansing your body energy

Imagine that you are coming out of a heavy, warm summer rain and you want to wick the water off your arms and legs and maybe your torso, too. With a slightly cupped hand and light motion, wick the imaginary water off your arms from your shoulders down to your hands, flinging it away into your surroundings. Do the same with your legs, front, sides, and back using both hands at the same time if you like.

You can also picture having fluffy pieces of dandelion seeds on your front and back that you want to brush off with the palms of your hand. Have fun with this exercise, imagining that you are ridding yourself of unwanted stress, tension, or cravings all while energizing yourself.

TECHNIQUE 9

Stop and Drop

Cravings have a mind of their own. Some wash over us at unpredictable times like waves in the ocean, and others arrive at specific times of the day according to the habits we have created. Once the habit has turned into an addiction, our mind can obsess about our next fix.

Breaking habits and addictions is very possible; many people have been able to do so. Knowing that cravings recur like ocean waves is helpful: just as waves ebb and flow, our wave of craving is bound to recede again. With this awareness, we know that although a craving appears, it will also disappear in time.

When we follow our cravings, we tend to focus solely on indulging and not on what will happen afterward. The urge to use, eat, drink, or do seems to be justified in our mind. Yet afterward our mind changes its tune toward guilt or shame. Having an awareness of this process can help you ride out your cravings.

When a craving appears, briefly stop what you're doing and bring to your awareness that the craving has the action of a wave that will rise at first and then disappear again—all you have to do is wait! Know also that with time the waves will become smaller and smaller.

Take five minutes to make a list of the consequences of indulging. While you are waiting for the craving to recede, explore how you would feel if you gave in to it. Make a list of what would happen on a physical or emotional level. Here are some questions you may ask yourself:

- What would the consequences be?
- Would I feel disappointed in myself?
- Would there be repercussions from my family and friends?
- Would my work suffer?
- Would other people be affected by my behavior?
- Would I feel that I broke my promise to myself?
- Would it seem that I have taken steps backward, despite the effort I put in previously?

- How would my body feel afterward?
- How long would it take me to recover?

And the most important question:

- *Is it worth it?*

Switching Your Brain On

The secret of getting ahead is getting started.
—MARK TWAIN

Overwhelmed: *Inundated, having hit the wall, overwrought, stressed out, at wits' end, end of the rope, burned out.*

Felicity has a frenzied life. Between her family, work, and household chores, she is often in overdrive. At times she even feels dizzy from the constant demands pulling her in all directions. When she feels particularly overwrought, she makes poor choices for herself. She eats too much, too fast, whatever food she comes across, and she drinks too much alcohol in the evenings. Felicity has made a habit of applying the Switching technique, as it is very effective in calming her down. Her thoughts stop racing, and she is able to make choices that are good for her.

When we get overtaxed mentally, emotionally, or physically, our body-mind will respond by "switching off" our conscious brain and our focused thoughts. This may happen after working too long, studying for an exam, or pushing our body beyond its physical limits. The same may happen when we feel stressed due to cravings or changes in our habits and lifestyle. We cannot think clearly, and we unwittingly shut down to give our body and mind a break. It feels like the thermostat needs to be reset before we can function again, before we can organize our thoughts and be able to make good choices.

When we are in that overtaxed state, the BodyTalk technique called Switching may come in handy. It can reset the nervous system to make it receptive and function at a more normal level. This, of course, will help us deal with cravings much better because we are more in charge, able to make better decisions, and choose healthier behaviors for ourselves.

HOW TO DO IT

In this technique, "Switching" means switching your stress off so you can turn your brain back on. Switching can reset the thermostat for stress in your brain, and it is easy to apply.

Make sure you take long, slow, and deep breaths while you do this technique and do not get uptight about doing it perfectly. Just go ahead—it's easy!

Follow the instructions 1 to 4 below in that order, not all at the same time. In other words, do them in sequence and not simultaneously.

1. With the index and middle fingers of both hands, lightly touch your closed eyelids. Put very gentle pressure on your eyeballs, about as much pressure as you would use if you were touching a baby bird. Leave your fingers there for one full breath cycle in and out. You may want to "look" downward, even though your eyelids are closed.

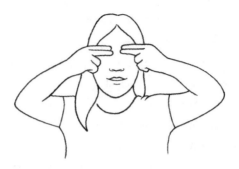

Two fingers over closed eyes

2. Place the thumb and index finger of one hand on the inside ends of both collarbones and wiggle your fingers for one slow breath cycle.

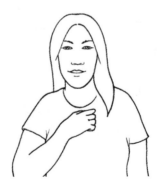

Wiggle your thumb and index finger on the inside ends of your collarbones.

3. Spread the fingers of one hand and gently tap on top of your head. You want your fingers along a line that roughly connects the top of your ears from one side of your head to the other. This is to ensure that you will tap on both the right and left sides of your head simultaneously. Tap with the pressure you would use on a baby bird and keep tapping for one whole breath. It does not matter how often you tap; just make it relaxing and gentle.

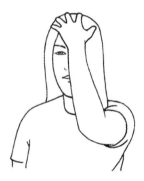

Tap the top of your head with one hand, fingers spread out.

4. Spread the fingers of one hand and gently tap on your breastbone. Use the same gentle pressure as before and tap for one whole breath.

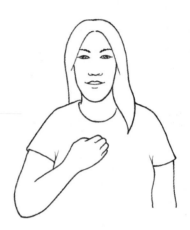

Tap middle of your chest with one hand.

Note: The last two steps are the same ones described in Technique 11, Sphenobasilar Balance.

Sphenobasilar Balance

Diane says, "When my system gets rattled, I make unhealthy choices for myself. The other day I almost got into a car accident and wanted to jump out of my skin. My first thought was to go home and make myself a stiff drink. What an unhealthy choice at that moment, and under such circumstances! The Sphenobasilar Balance technique made me feel better and I followed it with the Cortices balance. I felt renewed."

Eric hit the top of his head on the garage door a few months ago. Since then he has not been feeling the same, and he has had more of a struggle with his sobriety. Eric chose to try the Sphenobasilar Balance technique, and it turned out to be a very good way to bring him back into balance.

The sphenoid bone, also called the butterfly bone for its shape, and the basilar (occipital) bone are two of the important bones that form part of our skull. The connection between these two bones, the sphenobasilar (SB) junction, acts as an important hinge that allows brain fluid (cerebrospinal fluid) to circulate. Its movement is reminiscent of a teeter-totter, and it helps glands to work better and the "feel good" neurotransmitters to circulate.

The SB junction has a tendency to get locked, either after small accidents like hitting the top of your head on a door frame or getting hit by a ball or other object, or after emotional surprise or trauma. When we suddenly hold our breath or feel sudden distress, the locking mechanism of the SB joint can have a very dramatic, detrimental effect on our well-being. Being frightened or shocked or receiving bad news can result in a locked or stuck SB junction. We just do not feel right. We may feel low in spirits or struggle with brain fog, insomnia, or headaches.

When one feels off or distressed and vulnerable to cravings, performing a simple BodyTalk SB Balance can make all the difference. I have seen astonishing results in my practice with this technique.

I recommend using SB Balance when you feel that another technique is not working as well as you would like, or when a technique that used to work well has lost some effect. Having a functional SB junction will make all the techniques work better. It is like doing some basic wiring in your house: only then will the lights come on.

HOW TO DO IT

1. Breathe slowly and deeply.
2. Place the index finger of one hand between your eyebrows.
3. Put the index finger of your other hand under your chin, right in the middle in the soft spot.
4. Point that finger upward toward the top of your head.
5. Leave both fingers in place for two slow and deep breaths.

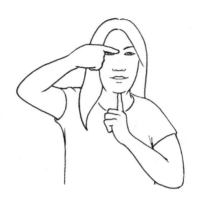

One index finger between eyebrows;
other index finger under chin

Tapping

Spread the fingers of one hand and gently tap on top of your head. You want your fingers on a line that roughly connects the top of the ears from one side of your head to the other. This is to ensure that you will tap on both the right and left sides of your head simultaneously. Tap with the pressure you would use on a baby bird and keep tapping for one whole breath cycle in and out. It does not matter how often you tap; just make it gentle and relaxing.

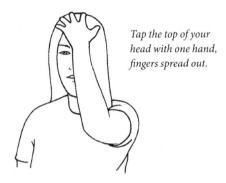

Tap the top of your head with one hand, fingers spread out.

Spread the fingers of one hand and gently tap on your breastbone. Use the same gentle pressure and tap for one whole breath.

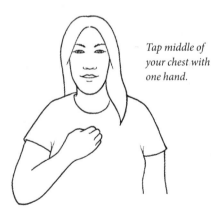

Tap middle of your chest with one hand.

Note: The last two steps were also described in Technique 10, Switching Your Brain On.

Healthy Habits

FILL THE VOID

*Just when the caterpillar thought the world
was over, it became a butterfly.*

—ANONYMOUS

Justin has had drinking problems for more than ten years. On many occasions his friends and family suggested he attend a rehab program, but for a long time he was not ready to address his issues despite the ill effects his alcoholism had on his work and private life. When he finally decided to quit, he made changes in his daily routine. Going to the gym every day gave him an activity to look forward to and a way to improve his mental, emotional, and physical health. Justin was pleased with how much better he felt!

•

Barbara enjoys her circle of friends and social events. Particularly in the summer she gets invited to outdoor events and cocktail parties. She became aware that the closer she was to the bar and food table, the more she was tempted to overeat and overdrink. She now chooses to chat with her friends at a good distance from the buffet. As an added benefit Barbara has noticed that she now pays much more attention to the conversations she is having, as she is not as distracted by the food and beverage offerings.

.

Most of us want to change our lives for the better, but often we don't know where to start. The best intentions falter as we, creatures of habit that we are, struggle to change our ways and get out of the rut we find ourselves in. Although behavior patterns can bring stability into our lives, they can also keep us in a negative state of mind and thus deaden our spontaneity. Having little or no spontaneity will reduce our joy in life to a dull and numbing compulsion.

The very first step in making a change is *deciding* to do something about the things you have been dreaming about. If you feel stuck in the traffic of your life and want to explore a side road with different and likely more interesting scenery, you can do so and benefit immensely from your decision. Not all side roads will have breathtaking scenery, yet by taking action sooner or later you will find a more fulfilling path. The most significant step is making the decision; everything else will follow from there.

After you have made the decision to change your life for the better, you will need to harness the powers that can assist you in making that change a reality.

HOW TO DO IT

Exchanging our limiting habits and behavior patterns for better ones takes just a little preparation. You are invited to engage in two brainstorming sessions; afterward you will be good to go at the spur of the moment whenever a craving hits.

Brainstorming session 1

What healthy habits do I want to develop to replace my detrimental habits?

Here is an example of a "healthy habit" brainstorming list:

- Go for a walk or bike ride.
- Feed the ducks or go birding.
- Sing or play an instrument.

- Research healthy foods.
- Learn to
  - sail
  - rock-climb
  - crochet
  - cook
  - garden

Now brainstorm your own list of healthy habits.

I am interested in developing these new habits:

_____

_____

_____

_____

_____

_____

_____

_____

_____

Brainstorming session 2

Next, choose one habit and brainstorm how you will go about establishing it. For example, imagine you are interested in learning to play the trumpet. Here is what your list might look like:

- I can call my friend Freddy and ask him to teach me.
- I can go to the local music store.
- I can read ads and look for a teacher.
- I can search the Internet for teachers or other musicians.
- I can find a musical instrument lending library.
- I can clean up my grandfather's trumpet.
- I can go to the second-hand store and find a used trumpet.

Now brainstorm your own list of how to establish your new habit.

This is how I will go about establishing my new habit:

_____

_____

_____

_____

_____

_____

_____

Learning to recognize early warning signs of our triggers is critical to creating healthy habits that stick. When we're aware of exactly when a craving will overtake us, we can develop a better strategy to counteract those cravings. Do you know what it is that triggers your addiction or craving? Is it something you hear, a feeling that creeps up, a sentiment that overwhelms you, a family holiday or anniversary? A good-luck celebration or bad-luck letdown?

Being aware of all of our triggers will help us recognize when we are in danger sooner, which in turn will help us engage in our healthy habits. The sooner we can act, the more secure our new healthy habits will become embedded in our nervous system. Remember, it's not enough to simply stop the detrimental compulsions, cravings, and old behavior. We also need to replace them and fill that void with new, positive habits and behaviors.

TECHNIQUE 13

The Secret of Service

*The only ones among you who will be
really happy are those who will have sought
and found how to serve.*

—ALBERT SCHWEITZER

Nothing will further your commitment to breaking
unhealthy habits like being there for other people.
Creating a sense of purpose in our lives by helping
others will shift our focus away from ourselves and
our busy minds that are constantly urging us to
"feed" ourselves and fill the big, empty space within.

Being of service to humankind on a regular basis
will help take our mind off the small circle of our own
existence and draw a larger circle full of interesting
people and new experiences. Understanding the
plight and needs of others can fill our void and make
us feel better about ourselves and more grateful for
what we have. There is a magical paradox in address-
ing others' needs and difficulties and extracting the
positive that lies within this experience for ourselves.

Psychiatrist and Nazi concentration camp survivor Dr. Viktor Frankl wrote several books about his dreadful experience during the Holocaust and about how having a purpose larger than oneself makes one stronger, more resilient, and happier. His life purpose was to help others understand that a person's search for meaning is our true quest, one that will truly satisfy the deep parts of our souls.

At the core of most spiritual and religious traditions is the notion that being of service to others is a direct path to greater contentment.

HOW TO DO IT

Make a list of ways you can use your interests and skills to serve causes you care about. Here's an example list:

- Practice Technique 7 and commit random acts of kindness. Help a neighbor, spend time with a child, visit a senior living facility, or become a Big Brother or Big Sister.

- Help out at the local food bank.

- Become a volunteer driver.

- Build houses for Habitat for Humanity.

- Become a member of a service club. Most service clubs have local and international projects.

- Volunteer at an animal shelter.

- Clean up around your neighborhood.

Let us assume that you have decided to be of service by helping to feed the hungry and you want to plan your next steps of action. You can start by breaking it down into two steps:

1. What do I want to do and what skills can I offer?

2. How am I going to go about it?

Here is an example:

1. *What do I want to do and what skills can I offer?*

   Brainstorming list:

   - Collect food from various places that donate it.

   - Cook in a soup kitchen.

   - Commit three hours a week to sort and hand out food items.

   - Clean tables and wash dishes at charity events that support a food bank.

- Assist a school program that helps students start food collections.

2. *How am I going to go about it?*

   Brainstorming list:

   - Call service clubs and ask if they have volunteer positions.
   - Go to the local homeless shelter and inquire if they need help cooking, serving, and distributing food.
   - Call the Salvation Army and ask if you can help in their soup kitchen.
   - Call the local food bank and ask if they need help.
   - Talk to restaurants and grocery stores and offer to transport unused food items.

Now make your list on the next page.

1. What do I want to do and what skills can I offer?

_____

_____

_____

_____

_____

_____

_____

2. How am I going to go about it?

_____

_____

_____

_____

_____

_____

_____

_____

TECHNIQUE 14

Pinch Away Cravings 1
THE MOUTH IN THE EAR

Sue loves good food a little too much. Too often she chooses to top off a meal with a rich, sweet dessert. Sue decided to try a variety of the techniques in this book to change her behavior and after a while, she realized that she no longer craved sweet desserts. She also noticed that she had smaller portions at mealtime, all with very little effort or restraint.

Like the foot, the ear is one of the reflex organs, meaning that every small part of the surface of the ear corresponds to an organ, body part, or mental state. By stimulating specific points on the ear—for instance, by massaging them or, as in the case of acupuncture, inserting a needle—you can enhance the function of an organ or balance your mental-emotional health.

There is one point that can help with the oral gratification needs involved in reducing certain cravings, such as quitting smoking, as well as the emotional needs related to overeating. Stimulating that point, sometimes referred to as the "million dollar point of auricular acupuncture," seems to be very effective in reducing oral gratification since it is the point that represents the mouth. By massaging the "mouth point," many of my clients have been able to reduce cravings. You can do so as well.

HOW TO DO IT

The mouth point is located on the outside of the ear just at the beginning of the ear canal. It is at the upper portion, the eleven o'clock position on the right ear and the one o'clock position of the left ear.

EAR ACUPRESSURE POINTS

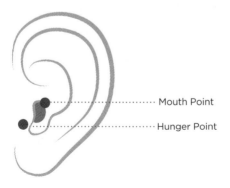

Mouth Point

Hunger Point

Take the eraser end of a pencil and use it as a massage tool to gently stimulate that point. Take care to *not* insert the pencil into your ear canal but to leave it on the outside and upper portion of it.

A point that can help to reduce hunger is located in front of the ear, in the soft part. You may want to massage that area as well. Acupressure always strives to enable harmony in the body, so you will not be able to "turn off" hunger completely. This technique will, however, help reduce unhealthy cravings.

TECHNIQUE 15

Pinch Away Cravings 2
RELAX YOUR BODY AND EMOTIONS

One of Emma's guilty pleasures was indulging in a candy from her childhood that was made in Great Britain. It was difficult to walk by the store that sold it without purchasing some. When she was tempted, she gave her ears a massage, being mindful of the areas on the ear that helped her relax. She noticed a big difference afterward, and she enjoyed the way her body felt. It helped her to keep walking past the store.

·

Acupressure points related to anger, depression, and anxiety can also be very helpful in making us more relaxed and mellow while lifting our spirits and easing our cravings. Massaging these points can greatly reduce the intensity of cravings and negative emotions, and therefore reduce the chance that you will give in to your unhealthy indulgence or behavior.

HOW TO DO IT

Lightly pinch your ears between your index finger and your thumb. Move along the outside of your ears from the bottom to the top, rubbing and massaging them. You may notice that some spots are tender and even exquisitely achy. Pay extra attention to those areas and work them a little longer and harder. You want to feel "good" pain but avoid intense or sharp pain. By doing this you have just given your spine a massage, and you may already feel a little more invigorated.

Now move to your earlobe. The science of auricular acupressure reveals that your earlobe represents your brain, face, jaw, neurotransmitters, and emotions. On the outside of your earlobe you will find a point that lifts your spirits. On the area of your earlobe closer to your face you will find the "anger point," a reflex point that can reduce the irritability that often occurs when we experience a craving.

Now massage your earlobes really well, and *voila!* —you just invigorated your brain and face.

The illustration below highlights the points that may be helpful to you. (A variation of this technique is also included in my book *Relieve Stress: 20 Quick Techniques*.)

EAR MASSAGE POINTS

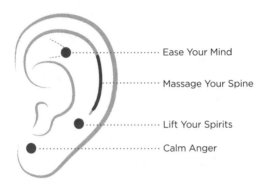

Ease Your Mind

Massage Your Spine

Lift Your Spirits

Calm Anger

TECHNIQUE 16

Zen Breathing

Sometimes Keisha felt agitated and restless, her mind and body focused on all the unhealthy ways she could soothe herself. Very soon after she started the Zen breathing exercise, she began to feel calmer. She could feel her thoughts shifting and her muscles relaxing. This technique allowed her to gain power over her temptations.

·

Breathing exercises are magnificent at slowing down our thoughts and gently increasing our energy level. Conscious breathing oxygenates our brain and our body.

This exercise is well known in Zen meditation practice, and it is very easy to do. It will help us when our cravings make us agitated and irritable. By focusing on our breath, our brain will be occupied with the act of breathing and will have a hard time continuing our previous harmful thoughts. We will likely feel more in charge of the choices we make after practicing Zen breathing.

HOW TO DO IT

1. Sit with a straight spine and breathe gently and fully in and out about five times. Relax your shoulders and the muscles of your face and body.

2. Now breathe normally and with awareness while counting every exhale. Once you reach five exhales, start over again from one to five.

3. Do this for five minutes.

You will inadvertently forget your count or find yourself at a higher number than five as your mind wanders off. Keep a sense of humor about this. Meditation and breathing exercises are not about achieving perfection but about observing what is happening inside your body and mind. Losing your count can become a part of the exercise; simply observe the process without judgment. This can be an excellent technique for calming your mind.

TECHNIQUE 17

Liver 3

Robin says, "I love massaging the acupressure point Liver 3. At first it is quite tender but after two minutes or so the pain dissolves. I can feel a release in my mind and my brain. It amazes me that I massage my foot and feel the effect in a completely different part of my body."

·

Naomi tends to massage the acupressure point Large Intestine 4, or Li4 (mentioned in Technique 1), as a default for dealing with sugar and food cravings, as it is so easy to reach and keeps both her hands occupied. She has found it very helpful, especially when a food craving is habitual, such as when she's watching a movie or at home in the evening. She also massages the Liver 3 point on the foot, which she says works even better.

·

When you are feeling grouchy, cross, and discontented, massaging the acupressure point Liver 3 may harmonize you and keep you from seeking your favorite indulgence.

Western medicine ascribes many tasks to the liver. It produces numerous proteins and hormones, it helps to digest our food, and it is the great detoxifier of our body. According to Western science, every liver cell is responsible for five hundred biochemical reactions; that is a magnificent undertaking. Chinese medicine and philosophy has a larger concept of what it means to "be" an organ: it correlates an organ with a consciousness and a mental-emotional task, an affiliation with other body parts, colors, seasons, and so on.

The consciousness of the liver is planning and organizing, and the emotions of irritation and anger "reside" within the liver according to traditional Chinese medicine. Considering that practitioners of ancient Chinese traditions believed the liver is the seat of the soul, we have even more reason to pay good attention to it and give it some tender loving care.

Massaging Liver 3 helps our body's detoxification process and may also decrease grouchiness. That is of great benefit to you, your life, and the people around you. The expression "liverish" for a dissatisfied mental state reflects our Western understanding of the liver being associated with anger.

Massaging Liver 3 can help you feel less irritable and therefore have more patience to make better choices for yourself when you experience a craving. It can also enable your body to eliminate toxins, not to mention ease the task of the liver while it's coordinating and performing those five hundred biochemical reactions.

HOW TO DO IT

Use your thumb to massage the area between your big toe and your second toe on each foot, about one inch from the web between them. There is a soft spot there, and it may be tender.

Give that point a good, hearty massage, following the usual rule: massage just enough to feel some tenderness but do not cause pain. If you feel tenderness on Liver 3, it indicates that this point is off balance and it will welcome some stimulation. Massage it for approximately three minutes on each foot and repeat a few times during the day.

Massaging Liver 3 can also improve our immune system, as the point is used in Chinese medicine to ward off colds, treat headaches, help with the blues, and lift pain in general, which in turn helps us stave off cravings that arise when we're in distress. Observe how you feel before and after massaging that acupressure point.

LIVER 3 ACUPRESSURE POINT

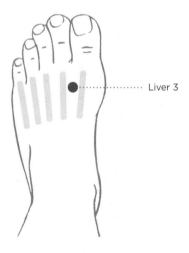

Liver 3

TECHNIQUE 18

Inversion Exercise
INCLINED TO DECLINE

After practicing an inversion posture, Tony felt lighter, as if stress had been brushed off his shoulders. He felt less worried, and the pressures of life seemed more manageable. The technique helped him put his thoughts and decisions into a better perspective.

•

This inversion exercise requires some physical dexterity. If you are able to sit on the floor and get up again without assistance, you may enjoy the benefits of this technique. Should you have any health concerns, please consult your physician before engaging in this technique.

This exercise can shift your mental outlook toward a more positive one. It improves the blood supply to your brain, giving it more oxygen and boosting your neurotransmitters, therefore helping you cope with cravings. You may even forget that you had cravings in the first place.

Inversions like this one are known to improve the functioning of your thyroid gland and can improve the health of your spine. All of these health benefits may allow you to make better choices for yourself.

HOW TO DO IT

Choose a clear space along a wall or against a closed door. Put a cushion on the floor and sit down on it with your shoulders against the wall. Now slowly and mindfully come down on the floor on one shoulder; then twist onto your back until you come to lie with your back on the floor (your buttock is on the cushion and almost touching the wall). If possible, extend your legs up the wall so that your body looks like the letter "L."

Now put your arms in a "T" position, take a deep breath, and relax. How do you feel? How do your surroundings look from this vantage point? Stay there for three to four minutes if you can and then slowly reverse your position. Take your time getting up while using the wall to steady yourself.

INVERSION EXERCISE

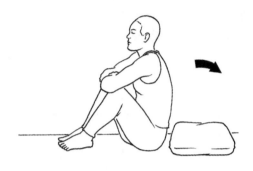

Slowly lower your back onto the floor and extend your legs up the wall.

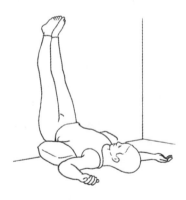

TECHNIQUE 19

The Artist's Way
CREATING A MANDALA

Creative focusing tools can help tremendously to bring attention to what we want and to fine-tune our internal vision for our life. Ancient cultures developed creative and powerful ways of aligning our thoughts and energies. One of the most popular techniques for this purpose in Eastern cultures is the mandala, a drawing or painting containing a circle representing the world or universe—or in this case, an aspect of our world. We can use the mandala to visualize our life, our surroundings, and our wishes and desires. It is a powerful tool that can help us focus on specific situations and the positive outcomes we desire. A mandala is comparable to a prayer with a creative and playful, yet nonetheless focused and serious, mind-set. Mandalas have been used in various contexts throughout history. You may be familiar with the sand mandalas that Tibetan monks created for centuries and continue to create to this day. You can easily make your own mandala and use it to gain insight into and set an intention for your own life situation. This exercise will tickle your creative bone while helping you to make positive changes in your life. It is not intended to be a piece of art but rather a reminder of what you wish for on your journey to reduce cravings.

Modern physicist Albert Einstein and the ancient mystics had something in common: they all knew that "energy follows thought." In other words, a thought is a real occurrence. From modern physics we know that energy can be measured as either a real particle of a material "something" or as a wave, like the rays of the sun or the light from your light bulb that enables you to read this book. Therefore, by this theory, thoughts have true substance, a cause and effect.

This exercise is easy to do, and you may get results either immediately or sometime down the road of your life journey. A word of caution to the mandala novice: be careful what you ask for, because you may get it. Be mindful and positive for yourself and others in your world. Make sure what you ask for is in harmony with everyone's wishes for a healthy and peaceful existence.

HOW TO DO IT

Take a piece of paper of any size and a lead pencil, pen, or colored pencils. Draw a large circle in the center of the paper, and then draw arrows from the circle pointing to the edge of the paper. It will look something like this:

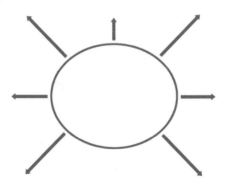

In the center of the circle write words or symbols that represent a state of mind that is free of cravings: for example, calm, peace, happiness, serenity. Be very clear with your choice of words. I would recommend that you actually add the words "free of cravings" in the center circle. You can use colors or images to illustrate this state if you like.

Outside of the circle, write words or symbols that represent the feelings or mental states that trigger your cravings or the cravings themselves.

Once you have completed these steps, quiet your mind and reflect on your mandala, focusing on the state you want to achieve that eliminates craving. You might fold up your mandala and carry it with you to remind you of that state when a craving strikes.

•

You can make other mandalas, including ones with words and symbols in the center that represent goals and desires that will contribute to your well-being. While you should feel free to reach for the stars, it is also important to set goals that you can actually realize.

Outside of the circle, write words or symbols for things that you do not want in your life and that might prevent you from realizing your goals. Remember to be mindful of the well-being of others.

Here is an example:

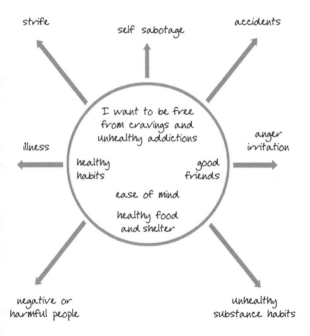

Trinity Breathing

Liza says, "I crave peace of mind. My mind loves to think, plan, organize, and improve. On and on it goes, playing pogo with my thoughts and coming up with new chores all the time; I call it spinning. It can be exhausting, as my mind just won't give me a rest. Like so many addictions, it is relentless in keeping me busy organizing my fixes—make new plans, improve the flow of things, fix the lawn mower, shop for nail polish, make a milkshake—all seemingly pressing tasks in my mind. From a saner perspective, the importance of these chores is rather questionable, of course! The Trinity Breath gives me a break, some peace of mind, and I can feel my nerve cells relaxing as my thoughts slow down, like a muscle resting after a heavy workout. The peace of mind feels delicious!"

•

The term "Trinity Breathing" was coined by Kate Cronin Haslach, a person who wears many hats in her life; she is a good example of living life to the fullest of one's talents. She swam the English Channel, is a fabulous professional cook, and authored *Fat Chicks Float Well*. Kate uses the Trinity Breath in her swim training and as a mind-calming tool for any yearnings that may pull her off-center. Having practiced Trinity Breathing for a long time, she notices shifts very quickly now. "The more you practice, the easier it becomes," she comments.

·

When we feel stressed, our breathing often becomes shallow, robbing us of good energy. Slowing down our breathing and taking deeper breaths can help to calm our minds and diminish our cravings.

This type of breathing is called the Trinity Breath because there are three balancing components to it. You can breathe the Trinity Breath wherever you find yourself: at your desk, in bed at night, while exercising, or when watching TV.

HOW TO DO IT

1. While slowly counting to five in your mind, inhale fully and mindfully, first filling your belly and then your lungs with air.

2. Hold that breath in for another slow count of five.

3. Slowly release your breath as you count from one to five, exhaling and letting go of as much air as you can.

After repeating the Trinity Breath for three to five minutes, check in with yourself: do you feel any different from when you started the breathing exercise?

Create Your Own List of Techniques

We are surrounded by people who deal with cravings, and they are all rich sources of knowledge and wisdom. To find out how other people abstain from their unhealthy indulgences, just ask them. Then use their answers to grow your list of techniques for reducing cravings and help you on your journey.

Here is an example of a question you could pose to a friend, coworker, acquaintance, or family member:

I have been thinking about how people curb cravings. If you ever crave any substance, food, or behavior, what do you do to change your mind and to reduce those cravings? Do you have any techniques? What do you tell yourself in order to get over your cravings?

I conducted my own interviews, and here are the answers I was given. If any of these appeal to you, add them to your list of techniques.

BRUCE:

I was craving "hard" when I was trying to quit smoking, and the evenings were the most difficult. One night I called a good friend and asked whether I could watch TV with her in the evenings when the cravings were intense. I knew I would feel too embarrassed to smoke at her house. I only had to call and invite myself to her house a couple of times, and it worked!

CANDACE:

I put a picture of a sumo wrestler on my fridge, and anytime I want to look for comfort food I see the picture as a reminder of why I want to eat a healthy diet.

NANCY:

I put up a picture of myself when I was younger and looked beautiful, twenty-five years ago. I look at it and it fills me with gratitude. It helps me to get over a moment of weakness.

CARLOS:

Changing my scenery is important. I may go for a walk or a car ride, go to a museum or out in nature—any positive change from my current location.

MEGHAN:

I brush my teeth and freshen up; that changes my mind-set! I also find that flossing my teeth relaxes me. It takes my mind off my cravings.

TIM:

My wife likes it when I crave because then I work outdoors and indoors, fixing what needs repair, cleaning, or chopping wood. Our place is in a much better state since I decided to quit drinking—and so is my mind! And as a good side effect, my wife is happy, too. "Happy wife, happy life," I say.

MARIA:

When I reach for a bag of chips, I often manage to stop myself. I say to myself: "No, you do not do that anymore. You have changed to a healthier lifestyle, and chips are a thing of the past." It feels as if I am stepping out of the person I used to be and into the new and healthier version of myself, and that reminder makes me feel better.

KYLE:

When I crave, I give a treat to my dog and take him out for a walk.

JULIA:

I remember when I was young: playing and using my imagination, I would be so focused on my joyful task that I would forget the world around me. Now, when I want to distract myself from my unhealthy urges, I find an activity that captivates me. It could be watching a movie I have been wanting to see, experimenting with watercolors, painting a piece of furniture, playing my guitar, or listening to my favorite music.

LEIGH:

Although I was not a heavy drinker, I was a habitual one. I wanted to reduce my drinking and felt for a long time like a failure because I had a hard time doing so. I started reading more about cravings and got some advice about changing my drinking patterns from a book called *Almost Alcoholic*. Then one day, out of the blue, I changed my drinking pattern. Instead of having wine after a long day at work, I had some fresh orange juice. I drank it out of a wine glass and celebrated the occasion. I felt so good! It was easy to continue from then on.

ELLEN:

When I need to get off my vice, which is sugar, I make a plan to change my life for six weeks. I look ahead and pick a time when I will have six weeks of limited distraction. I know that after three days my craving will almost vanish and I will feel much better. Having a large glass of water gives me a different "body feel" and helps in the process.

INGA:

When I want to quit, I tell myself that I cannot have what I crave for five days. So when my craving gets intense, I remind myself that five days down the road I can have what I want. Five days later, when I am happy about my success, I know I can keep going for a longer amount of time. That way I think I do not have to go "without" forever, and it makes quitting easier for me.

LIN:

When I am overcome with cravings, I watch a film or documentary of my favorite activity, which happens to be climbing. I watch those amazing climbers in nature, and it makes me feel so good that it takes my mind off my cravings.

TYREESE:

I get very irritable and anxious when I crave my substance of choice. I lose my sense of humor entirely. I realize I need a reality check. I put on a DVD of my favorite comedians, and even though I have heard them before I start laughing and keep laughing until my mind is in a different space.

JILL:

When I have a craving, I think of how I feel after I satisfy the craving. When I indulge, I feel emotionally guilty and bad about myself. I can feel churning in my stomach and my energy level drops. By connecting the craving with the feeling I have after indulging, I am often able to stay away from it.

KATHRYN:

I try to recognize the first warning signs of my cravings. With some practice, I can now recognize the beginning of a craving early on when I am still able to make better choices. The best thing I can do to deal with them is keep myself busy with something that makes me feel better and stay away from my substance of choice. I do a chore, clean, or run an errand and I feel I have achieved something. That makes me feel better and gives me a sense of accomplishment.

JOSH:

Dealing with cravings when I am quitting can be tricky. I tell myself that my usual behavior of choice is "not available" and "is not an option" and that I need to come up with plan B.

DONNA:

Large family gatherings are stressful for me. Big holidays can push me over the edge. As I have become more aware of the stress these situations cause and the poor choices I make for myself when under stress, I have learned that I need to plan ahead. Now I schedule some "me" time for after the event. I may set aside time to take a bath, go for a walk, or watch my favorite show. That way, when things get heated up at the gathering, I know I have an escape scheduled, and that takes my mind off the family dynamics.

•

I learned much from the answers I was given. I was both surprised and humbled at how willingly people answered my questions. In addition, it made me feel more connected to the people around me. I hope your interviews, along with the twenty techniques in this book, help you gain more insight into how you can cope with cravings.

Part II:

Theory and Background on the Techniques

The Zone

Ted Williams, the famous Red Sox baseball player, had an on-base batting percentage of over .480, which made him the all-time leader in his field. No doubt, he had practiced relentlessly since he was a boy; however, only someone in "the zone" can achieve such a feat.

"The zone" refers to a mental state of perfect balance, of being in the present moment. It means that all the fibers of your body, including your brain cells, are in absolute synchronicity. One body, one mind, one moment—in complete harmony. When we are in the zone, all of our systems are aligned, like a set of dominoes tumbling one after the other in perfect timing.

A person can be in the zone—and then out of the zone. Tiger Woods is a perfect example of this. For much of his golf career his mental state was in perfect alignment, his brain optimally focused and balanced. But once the stresses of life and fame caught up to him, he had a hard time staying grounded; his right brain and left brain were not in harmony. He was thrown off his game.

The same issue can arise with cravings. When we yearn or crave, we are not fully aligned in the present moment. We lean over, trying to reach something we have difficulty reaching and we become off-kilter, bending awkwardly until we fall.

The Power of Now author Eckhart Tolle tells us that all power lies in the present moment, not in the past or the future. The past is ruled by regret and the future is ruled by worry. Once we are fully aligned in the present, we are content; we function fully in the now; and there are no worries and regrets, only acceptance and appreciation of what is. We accept things the way they are without feeling the need to change them. We have no cravings!

How can we attain that level of equanimity? The answer is actually easy: by training our minds and thoughts, by practicing healthy exercise, and by feeding our bodies wholesome food. When we are on the path to becoming more in charge of ourselves, we move one little step at a time. We start our thousand-mile journey with the first step. We eat the "elephant" of the task one bite at a time. We will most likely get glimpses of what it feels like to be more at peace, to not be ruled by outward substances or compulsive behaviors.

A content moment here and a snapshot of equanimity there, and we will realize the benefit of this content feeling. It is bound to happen again and again as we become more and more intent on living a more authentic lifestyle. The mind- and body-balancing techniques in this book can help us experience moments of lightness, and after a while they can add up. When we falter, we get up and dust ourselves off, just as we did when we learned to walk. That is exactly how anyone can practice having more peace of mind: one small step after another. Practice makes perfect.

·

The Power of the Connected Brain

Life is not perfect, and most of us would agree that it is not easy either. There are those among us who have developed a calm attitude despite life's daily turmoil and trained their thoughts to reflect their steady outlook on life. We all know people who exude calmness. I am reminded here of the equanimity of the Buddhist or Taoist monks. Life is no easier for them than it is for the rest of us; however, they have arrived at a way of living and functioning that involves much more contentment. They seem to flow more gently through their daily ups and downs.

One way to become calmer while riding the roller coaster called life is by opening up our brain pathways to allow thoughts to flow more easily from one brain hemisphere to the other. In order to understand right- and left-brain balance, let us look at a simplified explanation of the central nervous system.

We have two halves of the brain (called hemispheres), and each of them is in charge of very different tasks and activities.

HEMISPHERES OF THE BRAIN

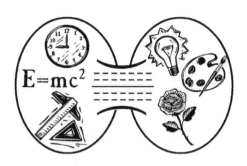

*Here are some tasks and activities of
each hemisphere of the brain.*

LEFT HEMISPHERE

- mathematics
- engineering
- bookkeeping
- punctuality
- organizing
- problem solving
- judging

RIGHT HEMISPHERE

- art
- listening to music
- poetry
- creativity
- relaxation
- appreciating nature

These two opposing sides of our brain are connected by a superhighway, the corpus callosum. When the traffic is moving smoothly on this superhighway, our thoughts are able to move easily from one side to the other. This facilitates the processing of thoughts and events and provides a sense of well-being and contentment. The challenge arises when the highway gets blocked and a traffic jam impedes the flow of nerve cell activity between the two sides.

We then feel off, unable to retrieve names, words, or phone numbers or to solve simple math problems. We become impatient because we feel overtaxed, and we make poor choices as the voice of reason eludes us. We may have studied sufficiently for an exam, but under the stress of taking the test we cannot retrieve the necessary information. We feel emotional and psychic pain. We want to soothe our unease, and we crave what the irrational parts of us think may lift our mood and help our plight. There are times when these choices are not only unhealthy but also dangerous for us. All these are examples of what can happen when a "connected" brain becomes "disconnected."

Let us now imagine a human brain functioning in a balanced fashion. The right, creative side of the brain would show considerable activity while the person is collecting flowers, humming a tune, or painting a picture. The left, logical side would show activity while the person is bookkeeping, using logic to make a better decision on a work project, or juggling all of his or her kids' homework and after-school activities.

When our brain functions optimally and all pathways are open, we are able to move quickly and easily from a task ruled by one side of the brain to another task ruled by the other side. We also experience perfect ease and acceptance of the present moment. When our nerve pathways are flowing well, we are able to call on any required areas of the brain without difficulty and master even complex tasks.

Unfortunately our lives rarely work like that; we function more from one hemisphere of the brain than the other. Some of us are talented mathematicians while others can easily create artistic works. Of course, we are born with a predisposition to function more on one side or the other, and we are also trained at an early age to favor one over the other. But when we spend too much time in one selective part of our brain, we lose the ability to take things in stride. We cover up the pain of discord, the difficulty of the mental traffic jam, by suppressing our emotions and indulging our senses in many ways. Before we know it, our indulgences are running us—and that's when they can turn into habits and addictions.

When we push down our pain, we lose touch with our positive emotions as well as our healthy sense of self. Our mind keeps longing for a fix. Once one craving is satisfied, it does not take long before we start seeking the next fix. Many times we do not even feel "satisfied." One soothed craving just leads to the next one.

The techniques in this book are meant to give you a glimpse of a balanced mental-emotional state, a sense of being in right-left brain harmony, even if just for a moment. Getting a glimpse here and there can move us forward and give us the confidence to overcome our challenges. Once we are connected to ourselves, our yearning can turn into acceptance, moderation, and discretion in how we satisfy our cravings. We are able to make choices that are wholesome and life affirming. All of us can achieve that state!

The Mechanics of Acupressure and the Meridian System

Acupressure and acupuncture make use of the body's meridian system, which was discovered a few thousand years ago by Chinese physicians. The meridian system is akin to the nervous system, but it is separate from the anatomical structures that we know in Western medicine.

Imagine twelve long, narrow "rivers" of energy flowing through either side of your body along prescribed paths. They are symmetrical, meaning they flow on each side of your body from head to toe and fingers, and vice versa. These rivers, or channels of energy, are important to our health in how they relate to our organs, other body parts, moods, and emotions.

We know that these channels, with about as many acupuncture points sprinkled on them as there are days in the year, carry an electrical charge that we can measure with an "ohmmeter," a device electricians use to measure electrical resistance. An acupuncture point conducts more electricity than its surrounding skin, and applying pressure to the point will help to balance this flow of electrical energy and create a self-healing response in your body.

Diagnosis in Chinese Medicine

In ancient China, autopsies were forbidden and medicine became the subtle art of "listening" to the body-mind. Chinese doctors were trained to be very observant and fine-tuned in the art of assessing their patients. There are three major ways that specialists of Chinese medicine find out what is going on in the body; namely, taking a careful history, taking the pulse in a way unique to this discipline, and looking at the tongue.

The first method is obvious and is used in any type of medicine. The patient reports as exactly as possible what he or she experiences in the body and mind; the aches and pains; and particular circumstances, patterns, and time frames of the complaints. The second method, taking the pulse, is a way of discovering what is going on inside the body by taking several pulses on both wrists. Chinese pulse diagnosis offers a window into the function of organ systems without blood work, lab tests, or imaging. It takes many years of study and practice to perfect the art and interpretation of "pulse diagnosis."

A number of years ago I traveled to China to study medical Qigong, an ancient system of postures, movements, and meditation techniques to create mind-body harmony. We visited a traditional Chinese medicine hospital and underwent Chinese pulse diagnosis performed by doctors on staff. The diagnosis established by these doctors who knew nothing about our medical history was astounding. They accurately described symptoms, imbalances, and illnesses in many of us.

When I learned the art of Chinese medicine at a course in Toronto, our teacher had us practice pulse diagnosis on other students. As I was feeling the pulse position relating to the heart, I noticed a "weak" pulse wave under the tip of my finger. The student, an upper-middle-aged man, confirmed that he had had a heart attack a couple of years previously. It seemed almost eerie to me then, but this kind of experience has become commonplace to me now after practicing Chinese medicine for more than two decades.

In addition to history taking and pulse diagnosis, Chinese medicine specialists practice the art of tongue diagnosis. The color, shape, and size of the tongue reveal much about a person's state of health and the condition of his or her specific meridians.

These three diagnostic tools give the doctors the information required to assess the meridian system and treat their patients. It is an eye-opening experience to have a doctor who is well trained in Chinese medicine and pulse diagnosis tell you about your state of health on a mental, emotional, and physical level without even knowing your name or your health history.

•

Famous Canadian neurophysiologist Dr. Bruce Pomeranz has conducted extensive research on how acupuncture affects the meridian system and found that potent neurotransmitters are released that benefit the body's healing system. This research is very important and meaningful; it does not, however, explain exactly why stimulating very specific acupressure points can help certain illnesses and support the health of an individual. Therefore, if you decide that you would like to explore using acupuncture or acupressure to treat a specific condition beyond the techniques in this book, finding a well-trained practitioner will make all the difference.

·

The Man in the Ear: Ear Acupuncture

Not all acupuncture is Chinese. It took a passionate and observant French physician by the name of Paul Nogier to discover the power of acupuncture points of the ear. You may have heard of foot reflexology, a system involving pressure points on the foot that reflect different parts of the body. The third technique in this book is based on foot reflexology. It turns out that the ears, like the feet, are "reflex organs." The story of ear acupuncture reads a bit like a fairy tale, albeit a true one, and when I first read about it as a sixteen-year-old, I was fascinated, as I still am many decades later.

Here is the abbreviated story:

Dr. Paul Nogier was a French general practitioner with a highly inquisitive nature. The intricate expressions and hidden physiology of the body fascinated him. He discovered that massaging certain points on the ears of his patients drastically reduced their back pain. At times he had to massage the ear quite hard, which, as you can imagine, could be rather painful. His patients, however, were thrilled because the ear massage often alleviated long-standing back pain. Nogier then started to use acupuncture needles on those specific points in the ear, a method that gave a gentler stimulation of the "back pain points" with good results.

The story does not end there. One day while he was holding the pulse of a patient, he touched certain active points on the ear and felt the patient's pulse shift under his thumb. It felt stronger or weaker in certain spots. He discovered that when there is a dysfunction or problem in a particular body part or organ, specific points on the ear are tender to the touch and, when stimulated, also shift the person's pulse wave. That was the birth of auricular medicine, by now a very sophisticated and refined modality practiced by medical doctors and practitioners around the globe.

What makes a point tender or "active"? Acupuncture points in the ear become active or tender when there is a problem in the body or mind. Active points carry a stronger electrical charge than the surrounding skin. The conductivity of electricity is higher in an active acupuncture point in the ear compared to the surrounding area, as shown using an ohmmeter. So whether you have back pain, are anxious or depressed, or have a sore tooth, your ear acupuncture expert can find certain points that have more electrical current flow across the skin in contrast to the surrounding area and that, when treated, can help you feel better. Auricular medicine has developed further into a sophisticated method for finding and adjusting underlying causes of health issues. It is particularly helpful for chronic illness.

*

The Benefits of Upside Down

Upside-down positions have been practiced by yogis for centuries. There are at least two benefits to hanging your head upside down, or "inversion," as it is called in yoga. I briefly mentioned the first one in Technique 18, Inversion Exercise: Inclined to Decline: it allows us to change the perception of the world we are used to in our everyday life.

Often when we can't untangle a mental-emotional issue, we are stuck in a certain gear. We can't move on or find a solution because our thinking repeatedly follows certain tracks in our brain, moving along the same nerve pathways and turning them into ruts. In order to unstick our thinking, it is very helpful to change our perception. Doing so can dislodge our habits of thinking so we use new nerve pathways and are able to find new views and solutions to a problem.

Changing our perception of the space we're in by "sitting on the wall" and looking up at the ceiling or sky frees up our brains. The very same thing happens with the problems we are facing. Suddenly more options open up before our very eyes, and we can see a variety of solutions that were unavailable to our previous, more limited thinking patterns.

There are biological advantages to the physical act of placing our head lower than our feet. Inverting our head allows gravity to increase the blood supply to our brain, providing good oxygen and nutrients. Also, our brain not only consists of the nerves folded into white and gray matter that most of us are familiar with; it also houses two very important glands, the pineal and pituitary glands (think of them as hormone factories), as well as higher control towers (the thalamus and hypothalamus, for example). The pineal gland is very important for our life rhythms, sleep and aging. In esoteric traditions, this gland is thought to be the seat of higher consciousness, our connection to the spirit within, or God. When we are anxious or depressed, we are disconnected from our inner being. Increasing the blood flow to and improving lymphatic drainage from the important glands in our brain helps with nourishment and detoxification, and *voila!*—the brain functions much better!

Our pituitary gland has the big task of keeping most of the other glands in our body stimulated and regulated. It regulates, for example, the thyroid gland and the adrenals and is important in maintaining blood pressure and producing oxytocin, the "feel good" hormone that helps us physically and socially bond with people. Oxytocin is also known to cause contractions during childbirth and is released during intimacy, making us feel close to our romantic partner.

The pituitary gland sits in a small, protected, bony cave in the brain that opens and drains at the top. Imagine a glass of water: you can empty it by drinking it with a straw, or you can turn it upside down and the water will flow much more freely. This is similar to what happens with the hormones of the pituitary gland. No worries, though—you will not dump too much of the good hormones at a time, as your body is too smart for that. Gravity will, however, improve the circulation of the hormones, provide more blood supply and drainage, clear more lymph, and tune up the gland's function.

You can see that inverting your body may help those good hormones go where they need to go: to their target glands and organs. This is another reason why inverting our body for a while will make us happier!

*

The Joy of Zen Breathing

We all know that breathing comes naturally, without any effort from our conscious mind. Thank goodness we don't have to constantly remind ourselves to take a breath! Breathing is one of our body's automatic functions, along with our hearts beating and the digestion of our food. No conscious effort is required to fill our lungs and rhythmically pump our hearts because the autonomic nervous system picks up clues and cues from our surroundings to modify the automatic activities going on inside of us.

The quality of our breathing is influenced by our deeper states of mind, and when we become anxious, stressed, and preoccupied, our breathing has a tendency to suffer by becoming shallower. Without being consciously aware of it, we may even take long breaks in between our in-breaths and out-breaths, thus further reducing the intake of life-giving oxygen.

Our autonomic nervous system, also called our involuntary nervous system, is crucial in influencing many of the automatic activities of our bodies. There are two branches that pull this internal function in different directions, like the two ends of a teeter-totter. The one branch, the sympathetic nervous system, can enable us to quickly burst into a thousand-yard sprint, running away from perceived danger, whereas the opposing branch, the parasympathetic nervous system, can help us relax, digest, heal, and turn on our immune system. Both systems are very important, as we need to be able to fight or flee (sympathetic) or heal and relax (parasympathetic) to maintain our bodies.

Anxiety leads to a state of stress, and our fight-or-flight mechanism runs in high gear. Modern-day stress and anxiety rarely prompt us to actually fight or flee, but they leave our internal systems revved up at high speed as though we needed to. This, of course, results in high levels of distress to our bodies, leading to a multitude of illnesses.

While we do not have control over our autonomic nervous system, we can influence it indirectly by making sure we exercise, relax, and restore ourselves through activities—or, rather, non-activities—such as gazing at the clouds, listening to music, laughing and visiting with people we love, painting a picture, watching old movies, or practicing the techniques in this book.

Breathing more deeply and deliberately can help our entire system to slow down, engaging the heal and relax system (parasympathetic) and increasing our oxygen intake. It can revive us, make us feel more alive, clear our thoughts, and energize us.

Paying more attention to our breathing cycle by slowing down our breath and being more mindful and conscious can have a calming effect on our mind by distracting us from its spinning and revolving thoughts. By practicing breathing techniques, such as the ones described in this book, we derive all the benefits of a formal meditation practice.

Ancient yogis also spoke of the positive effects of controlled breathing on our intestines because it causes our diaphragm, the breathing muscle, to contract more fully, thus gently massaging the insides of our abdomen. This improves blood flow, lymph drainage, nutrient uptake, and detoxification.

•

The BodyTalk System Explained: BodyTalk Cortices

BodyTalk and BodyTalk Access are energy medicine modalities developed by Dr. John Veltheim, an Australian chiropractor, acupuncturist, Reiki master, and philosopher.

BodyTalk is a very gentle yet profound way of balancing, aligning, and synchronizing one's body and its functions, thus improving the body's ability to heal itself. A powerful modality that can be learned by anyone, it is largely based on two concepts:

1. The body becomes "dysfunctional" when communication within or among organs, body parts, or the brain/mind becomes impaired. By finding the areas that need to improve and balancing their communication, the body can heal itself on its own.

2. The innate intelligence of the body knows exactly how it needs to address its healing and which problems should take priority. This means we can use BodyTalk techniques to bal-

ance and enhance the body's systems by tapping into the body's deeper wisdom. A practitioner uses neuro-muscular feedback as a tool to establish the type and sequence of balances used for each individual.

Any form of assault on the body, be it emotional, viral, or a physical injury, can potentially break down the sophisticated communication process in the body. Our bodies function as systems. The liver alone is responsible for five hundred chemical reactions, so it makes sense that it takes a good communication system to streamline the functions of the liver, let alone the entire body. Just as a factory production line would break down without a proper communication plan, so would the function of the body break down without constant communication within and among all its parts.

To understand this concept a little better, imagine going to a classical music concert. When you arrive early at the concert hall, you hear the musicians tune their instruments in the orchestra pit, and it sounds disjointed and inharmonious. During the performance, however, you hear beautiful music with the help of the conductor and musicians listening to one another and reading their sheet music. This is similar to what happens in the physiology of our bodies as communication among the various parts helps achieve harmony and balance.

The BodyTalk techniques Switching and Sphenobasilar Balance are stand-alone applications of BodyTalk and BodyTalk Access modalities. The hands are used as a focusing tool to activate the balance, and by doing so, the brain becomes unblocked, better able to function, and capable of paying attention to its needs. It enables better processing of thoughts, emotions, and other healthy brain functions.

For information about courses on this topic offered all over the world, visit the website of the BodyTalk Association: www.bodytalksystem.com.

·

Resources

Websites

Emotional Freedom Techniques:
www.emofree.com

International BodyTalk Association:
www.bodytalksystem.com

Women for Sobriety:
www.womenforsobriety.org

Books

Gach, Michael Reed. *Acupressure's Potent Points.*
New York: Bantam, 1990.

Gerber, Richard. *Vibrational Medicine: The #1
Handbook of Subtle-Energy Therapies.* 3rd ed.
Rochester, VT: Bear and Company, 2001.

Grabhorn, Lynn. *Excuse Me, Your Life Is Waiting: The
Astonishing Power of Feelings.* Newburyport, MA:
Hampton Roads Publishing Company, 2000.

Lipton, Bruce H. *The Biology of Belief: Unleashing the
Power of Consciousness, Matter, and Miracles.* Rev. ed.
Carlsbad, CA: Hay House, 2008.

Pert, Candace. *Molecules of Emotion: The Science
behind Mind-Body Medicine.* New York: Simon and
Schuster, 1999.

Tolle, Eckhart. *The Power of Now: A Guide to Spiritual Enlightenment.* Vancouver, BC: Namaste Publishing, 2004.

Veltheim, John. *The BodyTalk System: The Missing Link to Optimum Health.* Sarasota, FL: Parama, 1999.

Acknowledgments

I am grateful to the fabulous editorial and production team at Hazelden Publishing for their contributions and for giving me the opportunity to make these techniques available to more people. A special thank-you to MeeNah Pelland. I appreciate the effort and encouragement of my dear clients and friends who made this book possible.

About the Author

Katrin Schubert has dedicated her career to helping her fellow human beings heal their bodies, minds, and spirits with natural medicine. After completing her medical degree and a PhD in 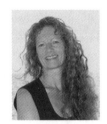 human genetics at the University of Hamburg, and receiving international training in England, the Czech Republic, India, China, Canada, and the United States, she opened her holistic health clinics in Kingston and Gananoque, Ontario, Canada. Katrin also has a science degree from Queen's University in Kingston. You can contact Katrin through her website: www.drkatrin.com.

About Hazelden Publishing

As part of the Hazelden Betty Ford Foundation, Hazelden Publishing offers both cutting-edge educational resources and inspirational books. Our print and digital works help guide individuals in treatment and recovery, and their loved ones. Professionals who work to prevent and treat addiction also turn to Hazelden Publishing for evidence-based curricula, digital content solutions, and videos for use in schools, treatment programs, correctional programs, and electronic health records systems. We also offer training for implementation of our curricula.

Through published and digital works, Hazelden Publishing extends the reach of healing and hope to individuals, families, and communities affected by addiction and related issues.

For more information about Hazelden publications, please call **800-328-9000** or visit us online at **hazelden.org/bookstore**.

Other Titles That May Interest You

How to Change Your Thinking
Hazelden Quick Guides
This collection of four eBooks applies the proven methods of Rational Emotive Behavior Therapy to challenge the irrational thoughts and beliefs that contribute to the debilitating effects of shame, anger, depression, and anxiety.

How to Change Your Thinking about Shame
Order no. EB4804

How to Change Your Thinking about Anger
Order no. EB4802

How to Change Your Thinking about Depression
Order no. EB4803

How to Change Your Thinking about Anxiety
Order no. EB4805

Craving
Why We Can't Seem to Get Enough
Omar Manejwala, MD
A nationally recognized expert on compulsive behaviors explains the phenomenon of craving and gives us tools to achieve freedom from our seemingly insatiable desires by changing our actions to remap our brains.
Order no. 4677; eBook EB4677

For more information or to order these or other resources from Hazelden Publishing, call **800-328-9000** or visit **hazelden.org/bookstore.**